ANTIANXIETY DIET

MAIN COURSE - 60+ Breakfast, Lunch, Dinner and Dessert Recipes for Antianxiety Diet

TABLE OF CONTENTS

purposes solely, and is universal as so. The presentation of the information is without contract or any type of guarantee assurance.

The trademarks that are used are without any consent, and the publication of the trademark is without permission or backing by the trademark owner. All trademarks and brands within this book are for clarifying purposes only and are the owned by the owners themselves, not affiliated with this document.

Introduction

Antianxiety recipes for personal enjoyment but also for family enjoyment. You will love them for sure for how easy it is to prepare them.

BLUEBERRY PANCAKES

Serves: **4**

Prep Time: **10** Minutes

Cook Time: **20** Minutes

Total Time: **30** Minutes

INGREDIENTS

- 1 cup whole wheat flour
- ¼ tsp baking soda
- ¼ tsp baking powder
- 1 cup blueberries
- 2 eggs
- 1 cup milk

DIRECTIONS

1. In a bowl combine all ingredients together and mix well
2. In a skillet heat olive oil

3. Pour ¼ of the batter and cook each pancake for 1-
    2 minutes per side

4. When ready remove from heat and serve

Serves: *4*
Prep Time: *10*   Minutes

Cook Time: *30*   Minutes

Total Time: *40*   Minutes

INGREDIENTS

- 1 cup whole wheat flour
- ¼ tsp baking soda
- ¼ tsp baking powder
- 1 cup apples
- 2 eggs
- 1 cup milk

DIRECTIONS

1. In a bowl combine all ingredients together and mix well

2. In a skillet heat olive oil

3. Pour ¼ of the batter and cook each pancake for 1-2 minutes per side

4. When ready remove from heat and serve

Serves: **4**

Prep Time: **10**   Minutes

Cook Time: **20**   Minutes

Total Time: **30**   Minutes

INGREDIENTS

- 1 cup whole wheat flour
- ¼ tsp baking soda
- ¼ tsp baking powder
- 1 cup mashed banana
- 2 eggs
- 1 cup milk

DIRECTIONS

1. In a bowl combine all ingredients together and mix well
2. In a skillet heat olive oil
3. Pour ¼ of the batter and cook each pancake for 1-2 minutes per side
4. When ready remove from heat and serve

Serves: *4*
Prep Time: *10*   Minutes

Cook Time: *20*   Minutes

Total Time: *30*   Minutes

INGREDIENTS

- 1 cup whole wheat flour
- ¼ tsp baking soda
- ¼ tsp baking powder
- 1 cup apricots
- 2 eggs
- 1 cup milk

DIRECTIONS

1. In a bowl combine all ingredients together and mix well

2. In a skillet heat olive oil

3. Pour ¼ of the batter and cook each pancake for 1-2 minutes per side

4. When ready remove from heat and serve

Serves: **4**
Prep Time: **10**   Minutes

Cook Time: **30**   Minutes

Total Time: **40**   Minutes

INGREDIENTS

- 1 cup whole wheat flour
- ¼ tsp baking soda
- ¼ tsp baking powder
- 2 eggs
- 1 cup milk

DIRECTIONS

1. In a bowl combine all ingredients together and mix well
2. In a skillet heat olive oil
3. Pour ¼ of the batter and cook each pancake for 1-2 minutes per side
4. When ready remove from heat and serve

Serves: *8-12*
Prep Time: *10*   Minutes

Cook Time: *20*   Minutes

Total Time: *30*   Minutes

INGREDIENTS

- 2 eggs
- 1 tablespoon olive oil
- 1 cup milk
- 2 cups whole wheat flour
- 1 tsp baking soda
- ¼ tsp baking soda
- 1 tsp ginger
- ½ cup cranberries
- ¼ cup molasses

DIRECTIONS

1. In a bowl combine all dry ingredients
2. In another bowl combine all dry ingredients

3. Combine wet and dry ingredients together

4. Pour mixture into 8-12 prepared muffin cups, fill 2/3 of the cups

5. Bake for 18-20 minutes at 375 F

6. When ready remove from the oven and serve

Serves: *8-12*

Prep Time: *10* Minutes

Cook Time: *20* Minutes

Total Time: *30* Minutes

INGREDIENTS

- 2 eggs
- 1 tablespoon olive oil
- 1 cup milk
- 2 cups whole wheat flour
- 1 tsp baking soda
- ¼ tsp baking soda
- 1 tsp cinnamon
- 1 cup durian

DIRECTIONS

1. In a bowl combine all dry ingredients
2. In another bowl combine all dry ingredients
3. Combine wet and dry ingredients together

4. Pour mixture into 8-12 prepared muffin cups, fill 2/3 of the cups

5. Bake for 18-20 minutes at 375 F

6. When ready remove from the oven and serve

Serves:	*8-12*
Prep Time:	*10* Minutes
Cook Time:	*20* Minutes
Total Time:	*30* Minutes

INGREDIENTS

- 2 eggs
- 1 tablespoon olive oil
- 1 cup milk
- 2 cups whole wheat flour
- 1 tsp baking soda
- ¼ tsp baking soda
- 1 tsp cinnamon
- 1 cup blueberries

DIRECTIONS

1. In a bowl combine all dry ingredients
2. In another bowl combine all dry ingredients
3. Combine wet and dry ingredients together

4. Fold in blueberries and mix well
5. Pour mixture into 8-12 prepared muffin cups, fill 2/3 of the cups
6. Bake for 18-20 minutes at 375 F
7. When ready remove from the oven and serve

Serves: **8-12**
Prep Time: **10**   Minutes

Cook Time: **20**   Minutes

Total Time: **30**   Minutes

INGREDIENTS

- **2 eggs**
- **1 tablespoon olive oil**
- **1 cup milk**
- **2 cups whole wheat flour**
- **1 tsp baking soda**
- **¼ tsp baking soda**
- **1 tsp cinnamon**
- **1 cup feijoa**

DIRECTIONS

1. **In a bowl combine all dry ingredients**
2. **In another bowl combine all dry ingredients**
3. **Combine wet and dry ingredients together**

4. Pour mixture into 8-12 prepared muffin cups, fill 2/3 of the cups

5. Bake for 18-20 minutes at 375 F

6. When ready remove from the oven and serve

Serves: *8-12*
Prep Time: *10*   Minutes

Cook Time: *20*   Minutes

Total Time: *30*   Minutes

INGREDIENTS

- 2 eggs
- 1 tablespoon olive oil
- 1 cup milk
- 2 cups whole wheat flour
- 1 tsp baking soda
- ¼ tsp baking soda
- 1 tsp cinnamon
- 1 cup kiwi

DIRECTIONS

1. In a bowl combine all dry ingredients
2. In another bowl combine all dry ingredients
3. Combine wet and dry ingredients together

4. Pour mixture into 8-12 prepared muffin cups, fill 2/3 of the cups

5. Bake for 18-20 minutes at 375 F

6. When ready remove from the oven and serve

Serves: *8-12*
Prep Time: **10**   Minutes

Cook Time: **20**   Minutes

Total Time: **30**   Minutes

INGREDIENTS

- 2 eggs
- 1 tablespoon olive oil
- 1 cup milk
- 2 cups whole wheat flour
- 1 tsp baking soda
- ¼ tsp baking soda
- 1 tsp cinnamon

DIRECTIONS

1. In a bowl combine all dry ingredients
2. In another bowl combine all dry ingredients
3. Combine wet and dry ingredients together

4. Pour mixture into 8-12 prepared muffin cups, fill 2/3 of the cups

5. Bake for 18-20 minutes at 375 F

6. When ready remove from the oven and serve

Serves: *1*

Prep Time: *5*   Minutes

Cook Time: *10*   Minutes

Total Time: *15*   Minutes

INGREDIENTS

- 2 eggs
- ¼ tsp salt
- ¼ tsp black pepper
- 1 tablespoon olive oil
- ¼ cup goat cheese
- ¼ tsp basil

DIRECTIONS

1. In a bowl combine all ingredients together and mix well
2. In a skillet heat olive oil and pour the egg mixture
3. Cook for 1-2 minutes per side

4. When ready remove omelette from the skillet and
    serve

Serves: *1*
Prep Time: *5*   Minutes

Cook Time: *10* Minutes

Total Time: *15* Minutes

INGREDIENTS

- 2 eggs
- ¼ tsp salt
- ¼ tsp black pepper
- 1 tablespoon olive oil
- ½ cup bacon
- ¼ tsp basil
- 1 cup zucchini

DIRECTIONS

1. In a bowl combine all ingredients together and mix well
2. In a skillet heat olive oil and pour the egg mixture
3. Cook for 1-2 minutes per side

4. When ready remove omelette from the skillet and
    serve

Serves: *1*

Prep Time: *5*   Minutes

Cook Time: *10*   Minutes

Total Time: *15*   Minutes

INGREDIENTS

- 2 eggs
- ¼ tsp salt
- ¼ tsp black pepper
- 1 tablespoon olive oil
- ¼ cup cheese
- ¼ tsp basil
- 1 cup red onion

DIRECTIONS

1. In a bowl combine all ingredients together and mix well
2. In a skillet heat olive oil and pour the egg mixture
3. Cook for 1-2 minutes per side

4. When ready remove omelette from the skillet and
    serve

Serves: **1**

Prep Time: **5** Minutes

Cook Time: **10** Minutes

Total Time: **15** Minutes

INGREDIENTS

- **2 eggs**
- **¼ tsp salt**
- **¼ tsp black pepper**
- **1 tablespoon olive oil**
- **¼ cup cheese**
- **¼ tsp basil**
- **½ cup feta cheese**

DIRECTIONS

1. **In a bowl combine all ingredients together and mix well**
2. **In a skillet heat olive oil and pour the egg mixture**
3. **Cook for 1-2 minutes per side**

4. When ready remove omelette from the skillet and
    serve

Serves: *1*
Prep Time: *5*   Minutes

Cook Time: *10*   Minutes

Total Time: *15*   Minutes

INGREDIENTS

- 2 eggs
- ¼ tsp salt
- ¼ tsp black pepper
- 1 tablespoon olive oil
- ¼ cup cheese
- ¼ tsp basil
- 1 cup tomatoes

DIRECTIONS

1. In a bowl combine all ingredients together and mix well
2. In a skillet heat olive oil and pour the egg mixture
3. Cook for 1-2 minutes per side

4. When ready remove omelette from the skillet and
    serve

Serves: *2*
Prep Time: *10*   Minutes

Cook Time: *15*   Minutes

Total Time: *25*   Minutes

INGREDIENTS

- 1 tablespoon olive oil
- 2-3 slices bacon
- 3-4 oz. breakfast sausage
- 2 green onion
- 2 eggs
- 2-3 oz. mozzarella cheese

DIRECTIONS

1. In a bowl beat the eggs with cheese and set aside
2. In a skillet brown the bacon
3. Add the sausage, onion and cook for 2-3 minutes
4. Add the egg mixture and cook for another 4-5 minutes

5. When ready remove from heat and serve

Serves: **2**

Prep Time: **5**   Minutes

Cook Time: **15**   Minutes

Total Time: **20**   Minutes

INGREDIENTS

- 2 slices bacon
- 2 eggs
- 1 tsp salt
- 2 burrito flour tortillas
- ½ cup cheese
- 1 green onion

DIRECTIONS

1. In a skillet cook bacon until crispy
2. In a bowl whisk eggs with salt and scramble in the skillet
3. Layer the eggs, bacon and cheese on a tortilla
4. Sprinkle green onion and fold

5. Cook in a skillet until golden brown
6. When ready remove from heat and serve

Serves: **4**
Prep Time: **5**   Minutes

Cook Time: **15**   Minutes

Total Time: **20**   Minutes

INGREDIENTS

- 4-5 pieces bacon
- 1 cup red onion
- 1 bell pepper
- 16-18 oz. hash browns
- 4 eggs
- 1 cup cheddar cheese

DIRECTIONS

1. Cook bacon until crispy
2. Add onions, peppers, hash browns and cook until soft
3. Whisk the eggs with pepper and pour egg mixture over the hash browns
4. Cook for 4-5 minutes

5. When ready remove from heat, top with cheese
    and serve

Serves: *4*

Prep Time: *15* Minutes

Cook Time: *20* Minutes

Total Time: *35* Minutes

INGREDIENTS

- 1 lb. bacon
- 4 eggs
- 1 cup white potatoes
- ¼ cup green peppers
- ½ cup cheddar cheese
- ¼ tsp salt
- parsley

DIRECTIONS

1. Cut bacon into thin slices and brown in a skillet for 5-6 minutes
2. Add potatoes slices, peppers, salt and cook until golden brown, when ready remove to a plate

3. Crack the eggs into the skillet and fry for 1-2 minutes per side

4. Spoon the eggs around the bacon and potato mixture

5. Sprinkle with cheese, parsley and serve

SIMPLE PIZZA RECIPE

Serves: **6-8**
Prep Time: **10**   Minutes

Cook Time: **15**   Minutes

Total Time: **25**   Minutes

INGREDIENTS

- 1 pizza crust
- ½ cup tomato sauce
- ¼ black pepper
- 1 cup pepperoni slices
- 1 cup mozzarella cheese
- 1 cup olives

DIRECTIONS

1. Spread tomato sauce on the pizza crust
2. Place all the toppings on the pizza crust
3. Bake the pizza at 425 F for 12-15 minutes

4. When ready remove pizza from the oven and
    serve

Serves: *6-8*
Prep Time: *10*   Minutes

Cook Time: *15*   Minutes

Total Time: *25*   Minutes

INGREDIENTS

- 1 pizza crust
- ½ cup tomato sauce
- ¼ black pepper
- 1 cup zucchini slices
- 1 cup mozzarella cheese
- 1 cup olives

DIRECTIONS

1. Spread tomato sauce on the pizza crust
2. Place all the toppings on the pizza crust
3. Bake the pizza at 425 F for 12-15 minutes
4. When ready remove pizza from the oven and serve

Serves: *2*

Prep Time: *10*   Minutes

Cook Time: *20*   Minutes

Total Time: *30*   Minutes

INGREDIENTS

- ½ lb. endive
- 1 tablespoon olive oil
- ½ red onion
- 2 eggs
- ¼ tsp salt
- 2 oz. cheddar cheese
- 1 garlic clove
- ¼ tsp dill

DIRECTIONS

1. In a bowl whisk eggs with salt and cheese
2. In a frying pan heat olive oil and pour egg mixture

3. Add remaining ingredients and mix well
4. Serve when ready

Serves: **2**

Prep Time: **10** Minutes

Cook Time: **20** Minutes

Total Time: **30** Minutes

INGREDIENTS

- ½ lb. bok choy
- 1 tablespoon olive oil
- ½ red onion
- ¼ tsp salt
- 2 eggs
- 2 oz. cheddar cheese
- 1 garlic clove
- ¼ tsp dill

DIRECTIONS

1. In a bowl whisk eggs with salt and cheese
2. In a frying pan heat olive oil and pour egg mixture

3. Add remaining ingredients and mix well
4. Serve when ready

Serves: *2*

Prep Time: *10*   Minutes

Cook Time: *20*   Minutes

Total Time: *30*   Minutes

INGREDIENTS

- 1 cup kale
- 1 tablespoon olive oil
- ½ red onion
- ¼ tsp salt
- 2 oz. cheddar cheese
- 1 garlic clove
- 2 eggs
- ¼ tsp dill

DIRECTIONS

1. In a bowl whisk eggs with salt and cheese
2. In a frying pan heat olive oil and pour egg mixture

3. Add remaining ingredients and mix well
4. Serve when ready

Serves: *2*

Prep Time: *10*   Minutes

Cook Time: *20*   Minutes

Total Time: *30*   Minutes

INGREDIENTS

- ½ cup leek
- 1 tablespoon olive oil
- ½ red onion
- 2 eggs
- ¼ tsp salt
- 2 oz. parmesan cheese
- 1 garlic clove
- ¼ tsp dill

DIRECTIONS

1. In a bowl whisk eggs with salt and cheese
2. In a frying pan heat olive oil and pour egg mixture

3. Add remaining ingredients and mix well
4. Serve when ready

Serves: **2**

Prep Time: **10** Minutes

Cook Time: **20** Minutes

Total Time: **30** Minutes

INGREDIENTS

- 1 cup broccoli
- 1 tablespoon olive oil
- ½ red onion
- 2 eggs
- ¼ tsp salt
- 2 oz. cheddar cheese
- 1 garlic clove
- ¼ tsp dill

DIRECTIONS

1. In a bowl whisk eggs with salt and cheese
2. In a frying pan heat olive oil and pour egg mixture

3. Add remaining ingredients and mix well
4. Serve when ready

Serves: **4**

Prep Time: **10** Minutes

Cook Time: **50** Minutes

Total Time: **60** Minutes

INGREDIENTS

- 4 chicken legs
- Juice from 1 lemon
- 2 tablespoons olive oil
- 1 tsp rosemary
- 1 tsp seasoning
- 2 garlic cloves
- 4-5 lemon slices

DIRECTIONS

1. In a bowl combine lemon juice, rosemary, olive oil, garlic gloves and seasoning
2. Toss the chicken with the marinade and let it marinade for 60 minutes

3. Place the chicken in a baking dish and 4-5 lemon slices along the chicken

4. Roast the chicken at 350 F for 40-50 minutes

5. When ready remove chicken from the oven and serve

Serves: **4**

Prep Time: **10** Minutes

Cook Time: **20** Minutes

Total Time: **30** Minutes

INGREDIENTS

- 1 lb. olive oil
- 1 lb. ground beef
- 1 garlic clove
- 2 tsp curry powder
- 1 tsp pepper
- 1 tsp salt

DIRECTIONS

1. In a skillet heat olive oil and sauté garlic until soft
2. Add the ground beef, pepper, curry powder and salt
3. When ready remove from heat and serve

Serves: *4-*
Prep Time: *10*   Minutes

Cook Time: *20*   Minutes

Total Time: *30*   Minutes

INGREDIENTS

- 1 tsp olive oil
- 1 lb. shrimp
- 1 tablespoon herbes de Provence
- 1 tsp salt

DIRECTIONS

1. In a skillet heat olive oil
2. Add shrimp, herbes, salt and pepper
3. Cook the shrimp for 3-4 minutes per side
4. When ready remove to a plate and serve

Serves: **4-6**

Prep Time: **10** Minutes

Cook Time: **8** Hours

Total Time: **8** Hours 10 Minutes

INGREDIENTS

- 2 lb. roast beef
- 1 cup beef broth
- 1 cup apple cider vinegar
- 1 tsp smoked paprika
- 1 tsp chili powder
- 1 tsp garlic powder
- 1 tsp cumin
- 1 tsp oregano

DIRECTIONS

1. In a bowl combine all spices together
2. Rub the beef with the mixture and let it marinade for 50-60 minutes

3. Place the beef into a slow cooker

4. Add broth, vinegar and cook on low for 7-8 hours

5. When ready remove from the cooker and serve

Serves: *4*
Prep Time: *10*   Minutes
Cook Time: *20*   Minutes
Total Time: *30*   Minutes

INGREDIENTS

- 1 lb. turkey
- 1 egg
- 1 tsp salt
- 1 tsp seasoning
- ½ cup red onion
- 1 tablespoon parsley

DIRECTIONS

1. Combine all ingredients together and mix well
2. Form 3-4 patties
3. In a skillet heat olive oil and cook each patty for 4-5 minutes per side
4. When ready remove from heat and serve

Serves: **2**
Prep Time: **5**   Minutes

Cook Time: **5**   Minutes

Total Time: **10**   Minutes

INGREDIENTS

- 1 cup broccoli
- 1 cup quinoa
- 2 radishes
- 2 tablespoons pumpkin seeds
- 1 cup salad dressing

DIRECTIONS

1. In a bowl mix all ingredients and mix well
2. Serve with dressing

Serves: **2**

Prep Time: **5**   Minutes

Cook Time: **5**   Minutes

Total Time: ***10***   Minutes

INGREDIENTS

- ½ cup pumpkin seeds
- 1 tablespoon olive oil
- 2 peaches
- 1 garlic clove
- 2 tablespoons parsley
- 2 tablespoons cilantro
- 2 cucumber
- 1 avocado
- 1 sesame sees

DIRECTIONS

1. In a bowl mix all ingredients and mix well
2. Serve with dressing

Serves: **2**
Prep Time: **5**   Minutes

Cook Time: **5**   Minutes

Total Time: **10**   Minutes

INGREDIENTS

- 1 tsp coriander
- ¼ cup olive oil
- ¼ tsp cardamom
- 1 cantaloupe
- 1 cucumber
- ¼ cup cilantro
- ¼ cup mint
- 1 cantaloupe

DIRECTIONS

1. In a bowl mix all ingredients and mix well
2. Serve with dressing

Serves: **2**

Prep Time: **5**   Minutes

Cook Time: **5**   Minutes

Total Time: ***10***   Minutes

INGREDIENTS

- 2 tablespoons lemon juice
- 2 tablespoons olive oil
- 2 cups snap peas
- 2 cups arugula
- 2 oz. prosciutto

DIRECTIONS

1. In a bowl mix all ingredients and mix well
2. Serve with dressing

Serves: *2*

Prep Time: *5*   Minutes

Cook Time: *5*   Minutes

Total Time: *10*   Minutes

INGREDIENTS

- ¼ cup olive oil
- ½ cup tofu
- 2 tablespoons lemon juice
- 2 cups romaine hearts
- 2 cups croutons

DIRECTIONS

1. In a bowl mix all ingredients and mix well
2. Serve with dressing

Serves: **2**

Prep Time: **5**   Minutes

Cook Time: **5**   Minutes

Total Time: **10**   Minutes

INGREDIENTS

- **2 Chioggio**
- **½ cucumber**
- **2 cucumber**
- **4 scallions**
- **2 chiles**
- **1 cups ricotta cheese**
- **¼ cup basil**
- **¼ cup mint**
- **¼ cup parsley**
- **2 tsp poppy seeds**

DIRECTIONS

1. **In a bowl mix all ingredients and mix well**

2. **Serve with dressing**

Serves: **2**
Prep Time: **5**   Minutes

Cook Time: **5**   Minutes

Total Time: **10**   Minutes

INGREDIENTS

- 1 cucumber
- 2 radishes
- 2 scallions
- 1 lb. snap beans
- ½ lb. greens
- 1 cup salad dressing

DIRECTIONS

1. In a bowl mix all ingredients and mix well
2. Serve with dressing

Serves: **2**

Prep Time: **5**   Minutes

Cook Time: **5**   Minutes

Total Time: ***10***   Minutes

INGREDIENTS

- 2 red bell peppers
- 2 spicy red chiles
- 2 garlic cloves
- 2 tablespoons red wine vinegar
- 4 oz. mozzarella
- 2 oz. salami
- 2 tsp marjoram

DIRECTIONS

1. In a bowl mix all ingredients and mix well
2. Serve with dressing

Serves: **2**

Prep Time: **5**   Minutes

Cook Time: **5**   Minutes

Total Time: **10**   Minutes

INGREDIENTS

- **1-piece ginger**
- **1 garlic clove**
- **2 tablespoons buttermilk**
- **½ cup Greek yogurt**
- **2 tsp rice vinegar**
- **2 tsp miso**
- **½ tsp onion powder**
- **½ tsp garlic powder**
- **1 lb. chicories**
- **1 tsp sesame sees**

DIRECTIONS

1. **In a bowl mix all ingredients and mix well**

2. Serve with dressing

74

CAULIFLOWER RECIPE

Serves: **6-8**
Prep Time: **10**   Minutes

Cook Time: **15**   Minutes

Total Time: **25**   Minutes

INGREDIENTS

- 1 pizza crust
- ½ cup tomato sauce
- ¼ black pepper
- 1 cup cauliflower
- 1 cup mozzarella cheese
- 1 cup olives

DIRECTIONS

1. Spread tomato sauce on the pizza crust
2. Place all the toppings on the pizza crust
3. Bake the pizza at 425 F for 12-15 minutes

4. When ready remove pizza from the oven and
    serve

Serves: **6-8**
Prep Time: **10**   Minutes

Cook Time: **15**   Minutes

Total Time: **25**   Minutes

INGREDIENTS

- 1 pizza crust
- ½ cup tomato sauce
- ¼ black pepper
- 1 cup broccoli
- 1 cup mozzarella cheese
- 1 cup olives

DIRECTIONS

1. Spread tomato sauce on the pizza crust
2. Place all the toppings on the pizza crust
3. Bake the pizza at 425 F for 12-15 minutes
4. When ready remove pizza from the oven and serve

Serves: **6-8**

Prep Time: **10**   Minutes

Cook Time: **15**   Minutes

Total Time: **25**   Minutes

INGREDIENTS

- 1 pizza crust
- ½ cup tomato sauce
- ¼ black pepper
- 1 cup pepperoni slices
- 1 cup tomatoes
- 6-8 ham slices
- 1 cup mozzarella cheese
- 1 cup olives

DIRECTIONS

1. Spread tomato sauce on the pizza crust
2. Place all the toppings on the pizza crust
3. Bake the pizza at 425 F for 12-15 minutes

4. When ready remove pizza from the oven and
    serve

Serves: **4**

Prep Time: **10** Minutes

Cook Time: **20** Minutes

Total Time: **30** Minutes

INGREDIENTS

- 1 tablespoon olive oil
- 1 lb. beans
- ¼ red onion
- ½ cup all-purpose flour
- ¼ tsp salt
- ¼ tsp pepper
- 1 can vegetable broth
- 1 cup heavy cream

DIRECTIONS

1. In a saucepan heat olive oil and sauté onion until tender

2. Add remaining ingredients to the saucepan and bring to a boil

3. When all the vegetables are tender transfer to a blender and blend until smooth

4. Pour soup into bowls, garnish with parsley and serve

Serves: **4**

Prep Time: **10** Minutes

Cook Time: **20** Minutes

Total Time: **30** Minutes

INGREDIENTS

- 1 tablespoon olive oil
- 1 lb. greens
- ¼ red onion
- ½ cup all-purpose flour
- ¼ tsp salt
- ¼ tsp pepper
- 1 can vegetable broth
- 1 cup heavy cream

DIRECTIONS

1. In a saucepan heat olive oil and sauté zucchini until tender
2. Add remaining ingredients to the saucepan and bring to a boil

3. When all the vegetables are tender transfer to a
    blender and blend until smooth

4. Pour soup into bowls, garnish with parsley and
    serve

Serves: **4**

Prep Time: **10** Minutes

Cook Time: **20** Minutes

Total Time: **30** Minutes

INGREDIENTS

- 1 tablespoon olive oil
- 1 lb. spinach
- ¼ red onion
- ½ cup all-purpose flour
- ¼ tsp salt
- ¼ tsp pepper
- 1 can vegetable broth
- 1 cup heavy cream

DIRECTIONS

1. In a saucepan heat olive oil and sauté spinach until tender

2. Add remaining ingredients to the saucepan and bring to a boil

3. When all the vegetables are tender transfer to a blender and blend until smooth

4. Pour soup into bowls, garnish with parsley and serve

Serves: *4*

Prep Time: *10*   Minutes

Cook Time: *20*   Minutes

Total Time: *30*   Minutes

INGREDIENTS

- 1 tablespoon olive oil
- 1 lb. lentils
- ¼ red onion
- ½ cup all-purpose flour
- ¼ tsp salt
- ¼ tsp pepper
- 1 can vegetable broth
- 1 cup heavy cream

DIRECTIONS

1. In a saucepan heat olive oil and sauté onion until tender
2. Add remaining ingredients to the saucepan and bring to a boil

3. When all the vegetables are tender transfer to a
    blender and blend until smooth

4. Pour soup into bowls, garnish with parsley and
    serve

Serves: *4*

Prep Time: *10*   Minutes

Cook Time: *20*   Minutes

Total Time: *30*   Minutes

INGREDIENTS

- 1 tablespoon olive oil
- 1 lb. mushrooms
- ¼ red onion
- ½ cup all-purpose flour
- ¼ tsp salt
- ¼ tsp pepper
- 1 can vegetable broth
- 1 cup heavy cream

DIRECTIONS

1. In a saucepan heat olive oil and sauté potatoes until tender
2. Add remaining ingredients to the saucepan and bring to a boil

3. When all the vegetables are tender transfer to a blender and blend until smooth

4. Pour soup into bowls, garnish with parsley and serve

PEANUT BUTTER SMOOTHIE

Serves: *1*

Prep Time: *5*   Minutes

Cook Time: *5*   Minutes

Total Time: *10*   Minutes

INGREDIENTS

- 1 cup soy milk
- 1 banana
- 1 tablespoon peanut butter
- ¼ tsp cinnamon
- 1 cup ice

DIRECTIONS

1. In a blender place all ingredients and blend until smooth
2. Pour smoothie in a glass and serve

Serves: *1*

Prep Time: *5*   Minutes

Cook Time: *5*   Minutes

Total Time: *10*   Minutes

INGREDIENTS

- 1 banana
- 1 cup ice
- ¼ cup blueberries
- 1 cup spinach

DIRECTIONS

1. In a blender place all ingredients and blend until smooth
2. Pour smoothie in a glass and serve

Serves: *1*
Prep Time: *5*   Minutes

Cook Time: *5*   Minutes

Total Time: *10*   Minutes

INGREDIENTS

- 1 cup strawberries
- 1 cup cranberry juice
- ½ cup orange juice
- 1 cup vanilla yogurt

DIRECTIONS

1. In a blender place all ingredients and blend until smooth
2. Pour smoothie in a glass and serve

Serves: *1*
Prep Time: **5**   Minutes

Cook Time: **5**   Minutes

Total Time: **10**   Minutes

INGREDIENTS

- 2 bananas
- 2 tablespoons cocoa powder
- 1 tablespoon maple syrup
- ½ cup peanut butter
- 1 cup ice
- 2 cups almond milk

DIRECTIONS

1. **In a blender place all ingredients and blend until smooth**
2. **Pour smoothie in a glass and serve**

Serves: *1*
Prep Time: *5*   Minutes

Cook Time: *5*   Minutes

Total Time: *10*   Minutes

INGREDIENTS

- 1 avocado
- 2 cups mango juice
- 1 cup orange juice
- 1 cup ice

DIRECTIONS

1. In a blender place all ingredients and blend until smooth
2. Pour smoothie in a glass and serve

Serves: *1*
Prep Time: *5*   Minutes

Cook Time: *5*   Minutes

Total Time: *10*   Minutes

INGREDIENTS

- 1 cup tomato juice
- ½ cup carrot juice
- 1 celery
- 1 cup spinach
- 1 cucumber
- 1 cup ice

DIRECTIONS

1. **In a blender place all ingredients and blend until smooth**
2. **Pour smoothie in a glass and serve**

Serves: *1*

Prep Time: **5**   Minutes

Cook Time: **5**   Minutes

Total Time: ***10***   Minutes

INGREDIENTS

- 1 cup strawberries
- 1 cup blueberries
- 1 cup yogurt
- 1 cup beet juice
- 1 cup ice

DIRECTIONS

1. In a blender place all ingredients and blend until smooth
2. Pour smoothie in a glass and serve

Serves: *1*
Prep Time: *5*   Minutes

Cook Time: *5*   Minutes

Total Time: *10*   Minutes

INGREDIENTS

- 1 banana
- 2 dates
- 1 cup Greek yogurt
- 1-inch ginger
- ½ cup coconut milk
- ½ tsp cardamom

DIRECTIONS

1. **In a blender place all ingredients and blend until smooth**
2. **Pour smoothie in a glass and serve**

Serves: *1*
Prep Time: *5*   Minutes

Cook Time: *5*   Minutes

Total Time: *10*   Minutes

INGREDIENTS

- 1 banana
- 1 cup coconut milk
- 1 tsp matcha powder
- ¼ tsp vanilla extract

DIRECTIONS

1. In a blender place all ingredients and blend until smooth
2. Pour smoothie in a glass and serve

Serves: *1*

Prep Time: *5*   Minutes

Cook Time: *5*   Minutes

Total Time: *10*   Minutes

INGREDIENTS

- 2 cups watermelon
- 1 cup soy milk
- 2 tablespoons honey
- 2 cups watermelon

DIRECTIONS

1. In a blender place all ingredients and blend until smooth
2. Pour smoothie in a glass and serve

THANK YOU FOR READING THIS BOOK!